Epilepsy in Special Population

Clinical Pearls

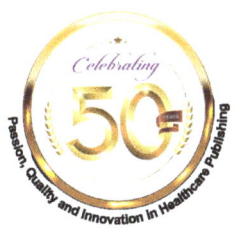

Epilepsy in Special Population

Epilepsy in Special Population
Clinical Pearls

Editors

Rajiv Anand MD DM
Director and Senior Consultant
Department of Neurology
BLK Super Speciality Hospital
New Delhi, India

Deepak Arjundas MD DM
Dip Neuro (London) FRSH (London) FAIMS FRCP
Consultant Neurologist
Vijaya Health Centre and Mercury Hospital
Chennai, Tamil Nadu, India

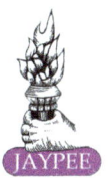

JAYPEE BROTHERS MEDICAL PUBLISHERS
The Health Sciences Publisher
New Delhi | London

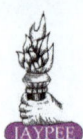 **Jaypee Brothers Medical Publishers (P) Ltd**

Headquarters
Jaypee Brothers Medical Publishers (P) Ltd
4838/24, Ansari Road, Daryaganj
New Delhi 110 002, India
Phone: +91-11-43574357
Fax: +91-11-43574314
Email: jaypee@jaypeebrothers.com

Overseas Office
J.P. Medical Ltd
83 Victoria Street, London
SW1H 0HW (UK)
Phone: +44 20 3170 8910
Fax: +44 (0)20 3008 6180
Email: info@jpmedpub.com

Website: www.jaypeebrothers.com
Website: www.jaypeedigital.com

© 2021, Jaypee Brothers Medical Publishers

The views and opinions expressed in this book are solely those of the original contributor(s)/author(s) and do not necessarily represent those of editor(s) of the book.

All rights reserved. No part of this publication may be reproduced, stored or transmitted in any form or by any means, electronic, mechanical, photocopying, recording or otherwise, without the prior permission in writing of the publishers.

All brand names and product names used in this book are trade names, service marks, trademarks or registered trademarks of their respective owners. The publisher is not associated with any product or vendor mentioned in this book.

Medical knowledge and practice change constantly. This book is designed to provide accurate, authoritative information about the subject matter in question. However, readers are advised to check the most current information available on procedures included and check information from the manufacturer of each product to be administered, to verify the recommended dose, formula, method and duration of administration, adverse effects and contraindications. It is the responsibility of the practitioner to take all appropriate safety precautions. Neither the publisher nor the author(s)/editor(s) assume any liability for any injury and/or damage to persons or property arising from or related to use of material in this book.

This book is sold on the understanding that the publisher is not engaged in providing professional medical services. If such advice or services are required, the services of a competent medical professional should be sought.

Every effort has been made where necessary to contact holders of copyright to obtain permission to reproduce copyright material. If any have been inadvertently overlooked, the publisher will be pleased to make the necessary arrangements at the first opportunity. The **CD/DVD-ROM** (if any) provided in the sealed envelope with this book is complimentary and free of cost. **Not meant for sale.**

Inquiries for bulk sales may be solicited at: jaypee@jaypeebrothers.com

Epilepsy in Special Population: Clinical Pearls / *Rajiv Anand, Deepak Arjundas*

First Edition: **2021**

ISBN: 978-93-90595-00-6

Contributors

EDITORS

Rajiv Anand MD DM
Director and Senior Consultant
Department of Neurology
BLK Super Speciality Hospital
New Delhi, India

Deepak Arjundas MD DM Dip Neuro (London) FRSH (London) FAIMS FRCP
Consultant Neurologist
Vijaya Health Centre and Mercury Hospital
Chennai, Tamil Nadu, India

CONTRIBUTORS

Abhilekh Srivastava MD DM
Consultant Neurologist
Fortis Hospital
New Delhi, India

Abhinav Gupta MD DM
Senior Consultant Neurologist
Sarvodaya Hospital and Research Center
Ghaziabad, Uttar Pradesh, India

Anand Diwan DNB (Neurology) MRCP (UK) Neurology SCE
International Diplomate American Board of Clinical Neurophysiology (Epilepsy), and European Board of Neurology
Consultant (Neurology) and Epileptologist, Narayani Hospital
Nashik, Maharashtra, India

Ashutosh Gupta MD DM SCE (Neurology) MRCP (London)
Consultant Neurologist
Navya NeuroCentre
New Delhi, India

Dhruv Zutshi MD DM
Consultant Neurology
BLK Centre for Neurosciences
New Delhi, India

G Butchi Raju MD DM (Neurology, AIIMS)
Consultant Neurophysician
Professor and Head, Department of Neurology
Andhra Medical College/KGH
Visakhapatnam, Andhra Pradesh, India

Himanshu Patel MD
Consultant (Neurology)
Jeevandeep Hospital
Anand, Gujarat, India

Jayanti Mani MD DNB (General Medicine) DM (Neurology)
Specialist Epilepsy
Epilepsy Fellowship (Cleveland Clinic, USA)
Consultant (Neurology), Kokilaben Dhirubhai Ambani Hospital
Mumbai, Maharashtra, India

Contributors

Joe Jacob MD DM (Neurology)
Consultant Neurologist
Amala Institute of Medical Science
Thrissur, Kerala, India

Joy D Desai MD DNB (Neurology)
Clinical Trial Office, Department of Neurology
The Jaslok Hospital and Research Centre
Mumbai, Maharashtra, India

Kamakshi Dhamija Verma MD DM
Consultant Neurologist
Kainos Hospital
Rohtak, Haryana, India

Kapil Kumar Singhal MD DM
Senior Consultant (Neurology)
Max Super Speciality Hospital
Ghaziabad, Uttar Pradesh, India

K Bhanu MD DNB (General Medicine) DM (Neurology) FMMC FRCP
Consultant Neurologist
Former Director and Professor of Neurology
Madras Medical College
Chennai, Tamil Nadu, India

Laxmikant R Tomar MD DM
Associate Consultant Neurologist
Sir Ganga Ram Hospital
New Delhi, India

Meenakshi-Sundaram MD DM (Neurology)
Associate Professor of Neurology
Department of Neurosciences
Apollo Speciality Hospitals
Madurai, Tamil Nadu, India

Moyinul Haq MD DM (Neurology)
Consultant Interventional Neurologist
EMS Hospital
Perinthalmanna, Kerala, India

Muneshwar Suryawanshi MD DM
Consultant Neurology
ClearMedi Health Care
Ghaziabad, Uttar Pradesh, India

Namita Kaul MD DNB
Consultant Neurophysician,
Vimhans Nayati Super Specialty Hospital
New Delhi, India

Neeraj Baheti MD DNB (General Medicine), DM (Neurology), Fellowship in Epilepsy (Sree Chitra, Trivandrum)
Consultant (Neurology) and Epileptologist
CIIMS Hospital
Nagpur, Maharashtra, India

Neethi Arasu MD DM (Neurology)
Neurologist
V Neethi Arasu Neuro Hospital
Madurai, Tamil Nadu, India

Praveen Kumar Yada MD DM (Neurology)
Consultant Neurologist
KIMS Hospitals
Hyderabad, Telangana, India

Pravin Naphade MD, DM (Neurology)
Honorary Consultant (Neurology)
Deenanath Mangeshkar Hospital
Pune, Maharashtra, India

Rahul Chakor MD DM (Neurology)
Consultant Neurologist and Epileptologist
Professor and Head, Department of Neurology
TN Medical College and BYL Nair Charitable Hospital
Mumbai, Maharashtra, India

Rajender Singla MD DNB
Associate Consultant
Sarvodaya Hospital and Research Centre
Faridabad, Haryana, India

Rajiv Anand MD DM
Director and Senior Consultant
Department of Neurology
BLK Super Speciality Hospital
New Delhi, India

Ritu Jha MD DM
Senior Consultant Neurology,
Sarvodaya Hospital and Research Centre
Faridabad, Haryana, India

Shruti Jain MD DM
Consultant Neurologist
Mind Mederi Neuro Care Clinic and Jaipur Golden Hospital
New Delhi, India

Suresh Reddy Challamalla MD DM (Neurology, NIMS)
Consultant Neurologist
Gleneagles Global Hospitals
Hyderabad, Telangana, India

Vijay Kumar Nandmer MD DM
Consultant (Neurology)
Gandhi Medical College
Kamla Nehru Hospital
Bhopal, Madhya Pradesh, India

VL Arul Selvan MD Dip NB DM (Neurology)
Consultant (Neurology)
Department of Neurosciences,
Apollo Speciality Hospitals
Chennai, Tamil Nadu, India

VT Ravi MD DM (Neurology, NIMHANS)
Consultant (Neurology)
Moulana Hospital
Perinthalmanna, Kerala, India

Preface

Epilepsy is one of the frequently encountered neurological conditions in clinical practice. It not only impacts the individual but influences the entire family. There are more than 12 million people with epilepsy (PWE) in India, which contribute to nearly one-sixth of the global burden. Seizures are unpredictable and adversely affect the patient's physical and mental health; increasing the risk of injury, hospitalization, and mortality. Besides, comorbid health conditions are common among PWE.

Incorporating available Indian guidelines for epilepsy management, this book collates key evidence and provides clinical tips to manage epilepsy patients in the busy life of practicing clinicians. Though there is abundant literature on epilepsy and different comorbidities the data is scatter and not presented in relation to Indian context. The primary motive of this book is to bridge the gap between evidence and practice and highlight clinical tips and pointers to enhance epilepsy management.

A clinician managing epilepsy does not just manage a single entity but manages the patient as a whole. This book thus, makes an effort to present key evidence and clinical tips for epilepsy management, as it would present in practical situations. Over the seven chapters the book addresses various common clinical situations. The initial chapters provide guidance on epilepsy management across various age groups, i.e., in children and neonates, in adolescents, and in elderly. The chapter on women addresses the most common issues of practical relevance while treating women with epilepsy. There are two chapters highlighting epilepsy management in two key comorbid situations, i.e., HIV and post-trauma, respectively. The final chapter addresses the management of emergency situation of status epilepticus. This book was curated with the help of enthusiast neurologists across the country and we were fortunate to lead this team. The key aspect of this book in our opinion is the "Clinical Pearls" section that provides practical tips and is an attempt to aid busy clinicians translate evidence into practice.

We hope the book serves its goal and provides some reference tips to ease your busy practice and enhance epilepsy management in the country.

Rajiv Anand
Deepak Arjundas

Acknowledgments

I would like to thank Shri Jitendar P Vij (Group Chairman), Mr Ankit Vij (Managing Director), Mr MS Mani (Group President), Dr Richa Saxena (Associate Director—Content Strategy), Ms Pooja Bhandari (Production Head), Ms Prerna Bajaj (Development Editor) and the publishing staff at Jaypee Brothers Medical Publishers (P) Ltd, New Delhi, India, for their work in completing this book.

Contents

CHAPTER 1	Seizures in Neonates and Children	1
CHAPTER 2	Adolescence and Epilepsy	4
CHAPTER 3	Epilepsy in Women	8
CHAPTER 4	Epilepsy in the Elderly	13
CHAPTER 5	Management of Seizures in the HIV Patient	18
CHAPTER 6	Management of Status Epilepticus	21
CHAPTER 7	Management of Post-traumatic Epilepsy	25
Index		27

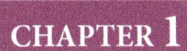

Seizures in Neonates and Children

NEONATAL SEIZURES

Neonatal seizures have an incidence of 1.8-3.5 per 1,000 live births. Neonatal seizures may exacerbate hypoxia ischemia induced brain injury. These changes in the brain may contribute to long-term neurological disability in some patients later in life.[1]

The challenge lies in differentiating neonatal seizures from several normal, poorly coordinated, neonatal movements.[1,2] Besides, there is lack of good treatment options.

CLINICAL PEARLS

- Neonatal seizures should be diagnosed accurately and treated aggressively.
- A rigorous workup to determine an underlying etiologic cause should be initiated quickly.
- When an inborn error of metabolism is suspected, discontinuing feeding may help improve the seizures and encephalopathy. Institute intravenous solutions and diet specifically indicated.
- Patients with seizures resulting from intracranial hemorrhage should have head circumference measurements performed daily. A rapid increase in head circumference may indicate hydrocephalus.

SEIZURES IN CHILDREN

Epilepsy is a common neurological disorder affecting 0.5-1.0% of children younger than 16 years of age. Several epilepsy syndromes have been identified in children (**Table 1**).[3]

Table 1	Focal epilepsy syndromes of childhood.	
Syndrome	Onset	EEG findings
Benign childhood epilepsy with centrotemporal spikes	Onset: 3–13 years Peak: 7–8 years	Bilateral asynchronous high amplitude, sharp and slow-wave complexes, with horizontal dipole, negative in centrotemporal regions and positive in frontal regions
Landau–Kleffner syndrome	Onset: 3–10 years	Continuous diffuse slow spikes and waves at 1.5–2.5 Hz occurring at all slow-sleep stages
Continuous spike-and-wave during sleep (CSWS)	Onset: 2–4 years	Infrequent spikes and waves; continuous diffuse slow spikes and waves at 1.5–2.5 Hz occurring at all slow-sleep stages, electrical status epilepticus in sleep (ESES)
Panayiotopoulos syndrome	Onset: 1–14 years Peak: 3–6 years	Interictal EEG with occipital spikes and multifocal, high amplitude, sharp slow wave complexes
Gastaut type	Peak: 8 years	Bilateral occipital spike-wave discharges that activate with eye closure and diminish upon eye opening

Comorbid disorders in children with epilepsy are categorized as neurological (cognitive impairment, migraine sleep problems), psychological [attention deficit hyperactivity disorder (ADHD), anxiety and depressive disorders] and physical (bone loss, weight changes, immunological disorders, dyslipidemia, hypothyroidism).[4]

There is a paucity of clinical trials of antiepileptic drugs (AEDs) in children.[5-7]

> **CLINICAL PEARLS**
> - Early and complete seizure control and EEG normalization is crucial for the prevention of developmental disablement in younger patients or of accelerated cognitive decline.
> - Focus not only on seizure control but also on early diagnosis and treatment of comorbid disorders.
> - Choose AEDs that best control seizures with minimal cognitive side-effects. AEDs such as levetiracetam and lamotrigine appear to have fewer cognitive side effects than old generation AEDs.

Continued...

Continued...

- Slow titration and using the lowest effective dose of AEDs is critical.
- Avoid polypharmacy.
- Treat comorbid neuropsychiatric disorders. Medications for ADHD and AEDs have drug interactions, e.g., methylphenidate may increase phenytoin serum levels. Carbamazepine may reduce methylphenidate levels.
- Because of the sedative effects of alpha adrenergics, cautious use is recommended in patients receiving sedating AEDs.

REFERENCES

1. Chapman KE, Raol YH, Brooks-Kayal A. Neonatal seizures: controversies and challenges in translating new therapies from the lab to the isolette. Eur J Neurosci. 2012;35(12):1857-65.
2. Panayiotopoulos CP. Neonatal Seizures and Neonatal Syndromes. In: The Epilepsies: Seizures, Syndromes and Management. Oxfordshire (UK): Bladon Medical Publishing; 2005.
3. Delphi B, Anilkumar AC. Self-limited focal epilepsies in childhood. Pract Neurol. 2018:64-8.
4. Wei SH, Lee WT. Comorbidity of childhood epilepsy. J Formos Med Assoc. 2015;114(11):1031-8.
5. Kessler SK, McGinnis E. A practical guide to treatment of childhood absence epilepsy. Paediatr Drugs. 2019;21(1):15-24.
6. Pellock JM, Carman WJ, Thyagarajan V, Daniels T, Morris DL, D'Cruz O. Efficacy of antiepileptic drugs in adults predicts efficacy in children: a systematic review. Neurology. 2012;79(14):1482-9.
7. Kim EH, Ko TS. Cognitive impairment in childhood onset epilepsy: up-to-date information about its causes. Korean J Pediatr. 2016;59(4):155-64.

CHAPTER 2

Adolescence and Epilepsy

INTRODUCTION

Adolescence is typically characterized by intense emotional and physical transformation and behavioral changes. Epilepsy is the most common neurological disorder of adolescence. Epilepsy may either have an onset during adolescence or it may be pre-existing epilepsy of childhood which continues in adolescence.[1-6]

INVESTIGATION

Establishing the correct diagnosis of both epilepsy and the specific epilepsy syndrome as well as any underlying cause is important (**Table 1**).

Table 1 Diagnosis of epilepsy and the specific epilepsy syndromes.[7]

Juvenile myoclonic epilepsy (JME)	• Presents at 12–18 years • Presents as bilateral, single or multiple irregular myoclonic jerks, chiefly occurring in the upper limbs, tonic-clonic seizures soon after awakening or absence seizure
Juvenile absence epilepsy (JAE)	• Occurs between the ages of 10 and 17 years • May have family history, photosensitivity • About 80% patients have generalized tonic-clonic seizures, often on awakening • Seizures occur exclusively or predominantly soon after awakening from sleep at any time of the day, with a second seizure peak during evening relaxation • Precipitating factors for seizures are sleep deficit, excessive alcohol or sudden arousal

Continued...

Continued...

Benign partial seizures in adolescence	• Onset is between 10 and 20 years, with a peak around 13–14 years, often seen in boys
• The patient has simple or complex partial seizures, which can be secondarily generalized. A cluster of 2–5 seizures in a 36–48 hours period may occur. The electroencephalogram (EEG) is typically normal or shows only mild abnormality
Photosensitive epilepsies	• These are common in adolescence, often seen in females, detected around 12–14 years of age
• The clinician must define the syndrome in which the photosensitive epilepsy occurs, such as JME or JAE
Reading epilepsy	• A rare, benign form of epilepsy, with strong genetic predisposition, occurs at 17–18 years of age
• The very characteristic motor/sensory aura helps in making the diagnosis: After reading for a period, abnormal sensations or movements occur (with full consciousness), involving the tongue, throat, jaw, lips and face
• If the patient does not stop reading, this aura may progress to a tonic-clonic seizure
Subacute sclerosing panencephalitis (SSPE)	• SSPE typically follows measles infection very early in life (under 2 years of age), presents in either in late childhood or in the teenage years
• Initially the patient may have subtle loss of intellectual ability but myoclonic jerks or more complex abnormal movements and dementia and eventual death
Epilepsy from cortical brain tumors	• It can occur at any age
• Neuroimaging of adolescents who present with partial seizures is important except in those who have characteristic benign partial seizures with a single seizure or cluster of seizures, no abnormal neurological signs and no recurrence

CLINICAL PEARLS

- Basic blood tests for full blood count, creatinine and electrolytes, calcium, and liver function tests should be performed. An EEG with photic stimulation should be obtained.
- Neuroimaging may be considered however, is not necessary in benign conditions.
- If possible, talk to the adolescent patient, friends and parents to get the accurate history about the episode of seizure.
- If substance abuse is suspected, then a urine specimen should be sent for toxicology testing.

TREATMENT

The treatment for epilepsy and the specific epilepsy syndromes are given in **Table 2**.

Table 2 Treatment or epilepsy and the specific epilepsy syndromes.[7]

Juvenile myoclonic epilepsy (JME)	• JME patients respond very well to sodium valproate • In nonresponders to monotherapy with sodium valproate, the addition of lamotrigine may be effective. Levetiracetam is also effective for treating the myoclonic seizures in JME • In women with epilepsy keeping the potential teratogenicity of sodium valproate and its subsequent negative impact on child development, levetiracetam/lamotrigine is preferred safe alternative
Juvenile absence epilepsy (JAE)	Sodium valproate, ethosuximide or lamotrigine
Benign partial seizures in adolescence	Treatment must be avoided unless there is a recurrence or unless there are particular reasons for treating
Photosensitive epilepsies	Adopt the appropriate treatment in line with syndrome identified
Reading epilepsy	Sodium valproate
Subacute sclerosing panencephalitis (SSPE)	
Epilepsy from cortical brain tumors	

CLINICAL PEARLS

- Characterize the syndrome and treat with the appropriate antiepileptic drugs (AEDs).
- Advise the adolescent:
  - To avoid sleep deprivation, alcohol, and substance abuse.
  - To avoid driving, potentially risky leisure activities such as rock climbing, horse riding, etc.
  - To avoid prolonged television (TV) viewing, playing video games and dancing in dark rooms with flickering/flashing lights in discotheques.
- Counseling is critical for parents and the patients. Include below points
  - Whether to continue with higher education.
  - Which jobs or careers would, and would not, be appropriate and when and how to apply for a job.
  - Methods of contraception and potential interactions between AEDs and the oral contraceptive.

REFERENCES

1. Wheless JW, Kim HL. Adolescent seizures and epilepsy syndromes. Epilepsia. 2002;43(Suppl 3):33-52.
2. Sheth RD. Adolescent issues in epilepsy. J Child Neurol. 2002;17(Suppl 2):2S.23-2S.27.
3. Besag FM. Modern management of epilepsy: adolescents. Baillieres Clin Neurol. 1996;5(4):803-20.
4. Engel J. Classification of epileptic disorders. Epilepsia. 2001;42(3):316.
5. Andermann F, Berkovic SF. Idiopathic generalised epilepsy with generalised and other seizures in adolescence. Epilepsia. 2001;42(3):317-20.
6. Koppel BS, Samkof FL, Daras M. Relation of cocaine use to seizures and epilepsy. Epilepsia. 1996;37(9):875-8.
7. Besag FMC. Chapter 42: Epilepsy in adolescence. Child and Adolescent Mental Health Services, London: East London NHS Foundation Trust (ELFT), Bedfordshire, and Institute of Psychiatry.

CHAPTER 3

Epilepsy in Women

INTRODUCTION

Women with epilepsy (WWE) pose unique gender-based problems pertaining to social and biological domains.[1-3] Epilepsy and antiepileptic drugs (AEDs) treatment affects sexual development, the menstrual cycle, and aspects of contraception, fertility, and reproduction.[4] The stigma associated with epilepsy and its consequences seem more detrimental in women as compared to men. They have more difficulty in getting married and sustaining a married life.[4,5]

POLYCYSTIC OVARY SYNDROME AND EPILEPSY

Epilepsy and AEDs influence the function of hypothalamic–pituitary–gonadal axis and lead to dysfunction of the endocrine system and change in reproductive hormones in WWE.[1-3] A recent meta-analysis of 11 studies demonstrated that the incidence of polycystic ovary syndrome (PCOS) in valproate treated WWE is almost 1.95 times that in other AEDs treated women.[6] Other drugs associated with the development of PCOS include oxcarbazepine and lamotrigine.[7,8]

> **CLINICAL PEARLS**
> - Valproate should be avoided in WWE in childbearing age.
> - AED best suited according to epileptic syndrome and without significant endocrine and teratogenic side effects should be chosen to treat WWE in childbearing age.

Continued...

Continued...

- If WWE are prescribed with valproate or other drugs that can increase the risk of development of PCOS:
  - Enquire about menstrual irregularity, weight gain, hirsutism, and galactorrhea.
  - In case of any positive history, perform ovarian imaging and hormonal examinations immediately.
  - Low dose valproate may be considered in resistant generalized epilepsy cases.
- New generation AEDs may be considered in women who develop reproductive endocrine dysfunction during treatment with the older AEDs.

CATAMENIAL EPILEPSY

About 35–40% of WWE have catamenial epilepsy.[6,9-11] Catamenial exacerbation is described in one-third of patients with drug-resistant focal epilepsy.[12] Women with catamenial epilepsy may experience a decrease in seizure frequency during pregnancy and menopause.[9,12]

CLINICAL PEARLS

- Ask WWE to maintain menstrual cycle and seizure diary and documenting seizure occurrence. A home video may help in diagnosis.
- In women with regular menses, the current treatment options is perimenstrual hormonal (e.g., progesterone) and non-hormonal treatments (e.g., clobazam or acetazolamide).
- In women with irregular menses, complete cessation of menstruation using synthetic hormones [e.g., medroxyprogesterone or gonadotropin-releasing hormone (GnRH) analogs] has been effective. All women with catamenial epilepsy may not respond to progesterone; it may benefit a subset of women with perimenstrually exacerbated seizures.
- The choice of drug depends on the type of epilepsy.
- Avoid sodium valproate. Choose levetiracetam, lamotrigine, zonisamide, and oxcarbazepine in younger patients.
- Follow-up both the mother and children for at least 6 years.

MENOPAUSAL WWE

At menopause, a complex multidirectional interaction occurs between sex hormones, seizures, and AEDs.[14] Anovulatory menses, possibly resulting in lower fertility, and earlier menopause can be seen in WWE.[14,15] Besides, menopausal WWE have an elevated risk for osteoporotic fracture due to the adverse effects of AEDs on bone metabolism.[14]

> **CLINICAL PEARLS**
>
> - WWE who have disruptive "hot flushes" may need to take hormone replacement therapy (HRT), at least for symptomatic relief and to allow adequate sleep. A combination of a single estrogenic compound such as 17-β-estradiol along with natural progesterone may be considered in these patients.
> - All patients should receive at least the recommended daily allowance of calcium and vitamin D.
> - Bone mineral density (BMD) can be considered especially in patients with long-term exposure to AEDs, particularly if the patient has other risk factors.
> - The new generation AEDs, i.e., lamotrigine, levetiracetam, and oxcarbazepine, are not associated with lower BMD.

PREGNANCY IN WWE

Pharmacokinetic changes occur during pregnancy as highlighted in **Table 1**.

Most WWE have uneventful pregnancies and healthy babies. But the risk of fetal malformations is increased when AEDs are used during

Table 1 Changes in the serum concentrations of new antiepileptic drugs during pregnancy.[13]

	Reduction in serum concentration
Lamotrigine	50–60%
Levetiracetam	40–60%
Oxcarbazepine	30–40%
Eslicarbazepine	NA
Topiramate	30–40%
Gabapentin	NA
Pregabalin	NA
Zonisamide	20–40%
Lacosamide	NA

(NA: not available)

pregnancy, especially in women taking polytherapy, or valproate. Infants exposed to AEDs in the antenatal period may suffer from neurocognitive and developmental impairment, low IQ or language problems.[16]

The important information for management of the lactating WWE is given in **Table 2**.

Table 2	Important information for managing lactating women with epilepsy (WWE).
Antiepileptic drugs (AEDs)	**Concentrations in breast milk and effects in infants**
Lamotrigine	Between 40% and 60% and correlates with the mother's dose
Levetiracetam	• Extensive transfer into breast milk • Breastfed infants had low levetiracetam serum concentrations, suggesting a rapid elimination of the drug. But no adverse effects were noted
Oxcarbazepine	• The milk/maternal plasma concentration ratio of the active metabolite of oxcarbazepine, licarbazepine (MHD), is 0.5–0 • No harmful effects in infants reported
Zonisamide	About 30% passes into the breast milk. Caution and close monitoring of the infant is advisable
Gabapentin	• Milk/plasma ratio of 0.7–1.3 is documented • Infant plasma concentrations ranged from 6 to 12% of the mother's plasma concentration • No side effects in breastfed children

CLINICAL PEARLS

- All WWE must undergo a detailed preconception evaluation wherein the need to continue AEDs, the ideal AED and dosage are reassessed.
- Folic acid supplementation to all women who could potentially become pregnant.
- Detailed screenings for fetal malformations need to be carried out between 14 and 18 weeks of pregnancy.
- The dosage of AEDs may have to be escalated in the second half of pregnancy in selected patients.
- The family should be provided detailed counseling and information on how to cope with the pregnancy, childbirth, and lactation.

Continued...

Continued...

- The new AEDs (except felbamate and vigabatrin) possess less favorable safety profiles compared to the classic AEDs.
- Wherever available, drug level monitoring of AEDs must be undertaken during different stages of pregnancy.
- Barbiturates and benzodiazepines pass into breast milk. New AEDs pass over into breast milk to varying degrees. Current data indicates that breastfeeding while taking new AEDs generally appears to be safe for the child.

REFERENCES

1. Amini L, Hematian M, Montazeri A, Gharegozli K. Comparing the frequency of polycystic ovary syndrome in women with and without epilepsy. J Family Med Prim Care. 2018;7(1):16-20.
2. Grzyb E, Kwiecińska P, Gregoraszczuk EL. Epilepsy, antiepileptic drugs and disorders of reproductive functions of women. Przegl Lek. 2014;71(10):544-8.
3. Bilo L, Meo R. Epilepsy and polycystic ovary syndrome: where is the link? Neurol Sci. 2006;27(4):221-30.
4. Luef G, Abraham I, Haslinger M, Trinka E, Seppi K, Unterberger I, et al. Polycystic ovaries, obesity and insulin resistance in women with epilepsy. A comparative study of carbamazepine and valproic acid in 105 women. J Neurol. 2002;249(7):835-41.
6. Joshi S, Kapur J. Neurosteroid regulation of GABAA receptors: a role in catamenial epilepsy. Brain Res. 2019;1703:31-40.
5. Begum S, Thomas SV. Women with epilepsy in reproductive age group: special issues and management strategies. J Assoc Physicians India. 2013;61:48-51.
7. Löfgren E, Tapanainen JS, Koivunen R, Pakarinen A, Isojärvi JI. Effects of carbamazepine and oxcarbazepine on the reproductive endocrine function in women with epilepsy. Epilepsia. 2006;47(9):1441-6.
8. Morrell MJ. Reproductive and metabolic disorders in women with epilepsy. Epilepsia. 2003;44:11–20.
9. Maguire MJ, Nevitt SJ. Treatments for seizures in catamenial (menstrual-related) epilepsy. Cochrane Database Syst Rev. 2019;10:CD013225.
10. Dupont S. Specific aspects of the management of women with epilepsy. Presse Med. 2018;47(3):251-60.
11. Kim GH, Lee HW, Park H, Lee SK, Lee SA, Kim YI, et al. Seizure exacerbation and hormonal cycles in women with epilepsy. Epilepsy Res. 2010;90(3):214-20.
12. Chalissery AJ, Murphy E, Mullins G, Widdess-Walsh P, Kilbride R, Delanty N. Recurrent catamenial status epilepticus: is it rare or an under recognized phenomenon in women with epilepsy? Epilepsy Behav Case Rep. 2018;9:19-21
13. Arne Reimer. New antiepileptic drugs and women. Seizure. 2014;23(8):585-91.
14. Sveinsson O, Tomson T. Epilepsy and menopause: potential implications for pharmacotherapy. Drugs Aging. 2014;31(9):671-5.
15. Harden CL. Polycystic ovaries and polycystic ovary syndrome in epilepsy: evidence for neurogonadal disease. Epilepsy Curr. 2005;5(4):142-6.
16. Reimers A. New antiepileptic drugs and women. Seizure. 2014;23(8):585-91.

CHAPTER 4

Epilepsy in the Elderly

INTRODUCTION

The elderly population is increasing globally. The prevalence of epilepsy in elderly in India is about 2.79% in individuals above 60 years.[1] But it has been postulated that the true incidence of epilepsy in elderly may be 2–3 times higher than these reported rates, because of difficulties in identifying seizures and diagnosing epilepsy in elderly.[2]

The elderly individuals are exposed to an increasing number of risk factors for seizures and epilepsy owing to their comorbidities and the presence of disorders that increase the risk of seizures.[2,3] Focal seizures are more common than generalized seizures in the elderly. Temporal lobe epilepsy is the most commonly diagnosed epileptic disorder. Absence seizures and status epilepticus are infrequent, but at times there may be a history of childhood-onset absence that has resolved, only to recur in later life with or without generalized tonic-clonic seizures.[2]

INVESTIGATIONS[4]

Approach	Features and tests
Careful history taking	• Obtain a moment-by-moment description of the event from a witness
	• Search for predisposing factors
	• Ask questions about sleep disorders, medications taken including over-the counter agents as they may lower the seizure threshold
Physical examination	• Thorough neurologic assessment
Initial laboratory evaluation	• Complete blood count
	• Electrolytes
	• Calcium

Continued...

Continued...

Approach	Features and tests
	• Magnesium
	• Phosphorus
	• Blood urea nitrogen
	• Creatinine
	• Glucose levels
	• An erythrocyte sedimentation rate
	• Liver function tests
	• Serologic tests
	• A chest radiograph
	• An electrocardiogram
	• When appropriate, serum drug levels and a toxicology screen should be obtained
Detailed cardiovascular evaluation	• Echocardiogram, Holter monitoring, and carotid Doppler ultrasonography
	• Acutely, computed tomographic scanning of the brain may exclude hemorrhage. When feasible, magnetic resonance imaging is the neurodiagnostic study of choice because of its sensitivity to infarcts and focal gliosis
Lumbar puncture	It is not routinely required unless the patient is febrile or has recently had a fever, meningitis is suspected, or the patient is immunocompromised
Electroencephalography	It can help to establish the diagnosis of epilepsy and classify the seizure type

CLINICAL PEARLS

- A detailed history must be obtained not only from the patient but also from an eyewitness, if available.
- The first step is to determine if the events are epileptic seizures or nonepileptic in nature.
- With recurrent falls and loss of consciousness, syncope must be considered as an alternative diagnosis.
- Visual auras may be epileptic or migrainous.
- Brain MRI is the most helpful neuroimaging study, although cranial CT scans may be performed in acute or emergency settings.

TREATMENT

Initial treatment must be monotherapy. The choice of a specific antiepileptic drug (AED) depends on the type of seizures and epilepsy, potential side effects (tolerability), physiological changes associated with aging, drug interactions, presence of comorbidities, need for rapid titration and cost.

The elderly population has altered physiology, low doses of AEDs are recommended in elderly patients with seizures or epilepsy. Besides, there are several drugs which may lower the seizure threshold and the patient must be asked about the use of such drugs (**Tables 1** and **2**).

CLINICAL PEARLS

- Start low, go slow.
- Modest maintenance dose.
- Assess renal, hepatic function, and plasma protein.
- Prefer monotherapy.
- Assess blood levels when indicated.
- Prefer nonsedating AED.
- Special attention to bone health and AED.

Table 1 Drugs which can lower the seizure threshold in elderly and cause seizures.[5]

Moderate risk	Intermediate risk	Low risk
Chlorpromazine	Other antipsychotic agents	• Risperidone • Quetiapine
Clozapine	Cyclic antidepressants	SSRIs, MAOI
Olanzapine	Bupropion	Local anesthetics
Clomipramine	Methylphenidate	Antivirals
Maprotiline	Tramadol	• Other antibiotics • Quinolones
Pethidine	• Beta-lactam antibiotics Isoniazid Metronidazole • Theophylline, aminophylline	Beta-blockers

(MAOI: monoamine oxidase inhibitors; SSRIs: selective serotonin reuptake inhibitors)

Table 2. Advantages and disadvantages of using antiepileptic drugs (AEDs) in the elderly.[5]

AEDs	Advantages	Disadvantages
Carbamazepine	Good efficacy	• Narrow therapeutic index • Hepatic enzyme inducer, rash • Hyponatremia
Valproate	Broad spectrum, IV, rapid titration	Causes weight gain, encephalopathy, tremor, urinary retention, arrhythmia
Gabapentin	Rapid titration, few AEs, no drug interaction	Limited efficacy, multiple-daily dosing, renal clearance
Pregabalin	No drug interaction	Somnolence, weight gain
Lamotrigine	Broad spectrum, no cognitive AEs, psychotropic effect	Titration is complex, rash
Levetiracetam	Good efficacy, broad spectrum, rapid titration, IV, no interaction, no cognitive AEs	Psychiatric dysfunction, dose adjustment required based on the GFR
Oxcarbazepine	Good efficacy, better PK/AE profile than carbamazepine	Rash, hyponatremia
Topiramate	Good efficacy, broad spectrum, low PK interaction	Impaired cognitive, glaucoma, weight loss, renal stone
Zonisamide	Good efficacy, broad spectrum, less risk of PK interaction, once-daily dosing	Affects cognition, cognitive AEs, weight loss, renal stone
Lacosamide	High efficacy, rapid titration, IV, no PK interaction, low cognitive SE	Dizziness, arrhythmia
Perampanel	Broad spectrum, long half-life	Somnolence, dizziness

(AEs: adverse effects; IV: intravenous; GFR: glomerular filtration rate; PK: pharmacokinetic; SE: status epilepticus)

Epilepsy surgery is less often performed in the elderly since they respond well to AEDs.[6-10]

CLINICAL PEARLS

- Carefully consider the comorbid disorders in the elderly patient so that the AED can be chosen appropriately.
- Choose drugs (such as levetiracetam, lamotrigine) with a good tolerability profile so that adherence to treatment can be ensured.
- Avoid polytherapy.
- Consider therapeutic drug monitoring when indicated.

REFERENCES

1. Beghi E, Giussani G. Aging and the epidemiology of epilepsy. Neuroepidemiology. 2018;51:216-23.
2. Acharya JN, Acharya VJ. Epilepsy in the elderly: special considerations and challenges. Ann Indian Acad Neurol. 2014;17(Suppl 1):S18-26.
3. Kaur U, Chauhan I, Gambhir IS, Chakrabarti SS. Antiepileptic drug therapy in the elderly: a clinical pharmacological review. Acta Neurol Belg. 2019;119(2):163-73.
4. Vélez L. Seizure disorders in the elderly. Am Fam Physician. 2003;67:325-32.
5. Sang Kun Lee. Epilepsy in the elderly: treatment and consideration of comorbid diseases. J Epilepsy Res. 2019;9(1):27-35.
6. McLachlan RS, Chovaz CJ, Blume WT, Girvin JP. Temporal lobectomy for intractable epilepsy in patients over age 45 years. Neurology. 1992;42(3 Pt 1):662-5.
7. Sirven JI, Malamut BL, O'Connor M, Sperling MR. Temporal lobectomy in older versus younger adults. Neurology. 2000;54:2166-70.
8. Boling W, Andermann F, Reutens D, Dubeau F, Caporicci L, Olivier A. Surgery for temporal lobe epilepsy in older patients. J Neurosurg. 2001;95:242-8.
9. Grivas A, Schramm J, Kral T, von Lehe M, Helmstaedter C, Elger C, et al. Surgical treatment for refractory temporal lobe epilepsy in the elderly: seizure outcome and neuropsychological sequels compared with a younger cohort. Epilepsia. 2006;47:1364-72.
10. Tellez-Zenteno JF, Sadanand V, Riesberry M, Robinson CA, Ogieglo L, Masiowski P, et al. Epilepsy surgery in the elderly: An unusual case of a 75 year old man with recurrent status epilepticus. Epileptic Disord. 2009;11:144-9.

CHAPTER 5

Management of Seizures in the HIV Patient

INTRODUCTION

Seizures and epilepsy are important central nervous system (CNS) complications of human immunodeficiency virus (HIV) infection.[1] An incidence of seizures of about 11% was observed in HIV-infected patients. New-onset seizures were observed in 4% of AIDS patients.[1] Seizures in HIV patients have a high recurrence rate.[2] In the majority of patients, seizures are of the generalized type.

INVESTIGATION

A thorough evaluation of the HIV patient is critical to investigate the underlying cause for the seizure.[3] Electroencephalography (EEG) is required for evaluating seizure recurrence risk and to distinguish encephalopathy from nonconvulsive status epilepticus in patients with persistent obtundation.[3]

TREATMENT

The management of seizures in the HIV patient can be considered in two phases namely: (1) acute to control the seizures immediately; and (2) subsequent management after control of the acute seizures.

Patient evaluations for the seizure type and comorbid medical conditions are essential to help make the decision about the appropriate antiepileptic drugs (AEDs) for the patient (**Tables 1** and **2**).

The favored AEDs for use in HIV+ patients are levetiracetam, lacosamide, gabapentin, pregabalin (**Table 3**).[3]

Table 1. Drug interactions of antiepileptic drugs (AEDs) and HAART drugs.

AED	Drug interactions
Lamotrigine	Lopinavir/ritonavir and atazanavir/ritonavir both resulted in decreased bioavailability of lamotrigine
Carbamazepine and phenytoin	Reduced half-life of the NNRTI nevirapine
Oxcarbazepine	• No significant pharmacokinetic interaction with ARV drugs • However, it should be used with caution in any patient with HIV+ and hyponatremia as it can exacerbate hyponatremia
Clobazam	Neurotoxicity occurs from increased concentrations of clobazam when coadministered with the NNRTI etravirine

(ARV: antiretroviral; HAART: highly active antiretroviral therapy; NNRTI: non-nucleoside reverse transcriptase inhibitor)

Table 2. Dose adjustment in AEDs: HAART interactions.[4]

AED	HAART	Dose adjustment
Phenytoin	Lopinavir/ritonavir	Increase HAART 50%
Valproic acid	• Zidovudine • Efavirenz	• Decrease HAART dose • No dose adjustment
Lamotrigine	• Ritonavir/atazanavir • Raltegravir/atazanavir	• Increase AED by 50% • No AED adjustment
Midazolam	Raltegravir	No AED adjustment

(HAART: highly active antiretroviral therapy; AEDs: antiepileptic drugs)

Table 3. Antiepileptic drugs (AEDs) for human immunodeficiency virus (HIV) patients.

AED	Features
Levetiracetam	• Most commonly prescribed • It has a broad spectrum of activity • Its metabolism does not involve the enzymes of the cytochrome P450 system • Levetiracetam is almost entirely renally cleared • In patients with documented renal disease it may require dosage adjustment for impaired creatinine clearance

Continued...

Continued...

Lacosamide	Electrocardiogram (ECG) should be performed prior to administration to screen for possible cardiac conduction defects
Gabapentin	Gabapentin is almost entirely renally cleared thus in patients with documented renal disease it may require dosage adjustment for impaired creatinine clearance
Pregabalin	Pregabalin is almost entirely renally cleared thus in patients with documented renal disease it may require dosage adjustment for impaired creatinine clearance

CLINICAL PEARLS

- Prompt diagnosis of seizure type is important.
- Investigate for the underlying cause of seizures with the appropriate battery of tests.
- Prompt treatment of identified infections is critical.
- Evaluate for the presence of organ dysfunction and comorbid conditions.
- When deciding upon the treatment options consider the risk of AED-antiretroviral (ARV) interactions.
- Avoid enzyme-inducing AEDs (older generation AEDs such as primidone, phenytoin, phenobarbital, and carbamazepine) in people on ARV regimens that include protease inhibitors or non-nucleoside reverse transcriptase inhibitors as pharmacokinetic interactions can lead to virologic failure.
- Be alert for drug related side effects which may worsen or can be confused with symptoms of HIV and/or epilepsy.
- In patients with drug resistant epilepsy, evaluate if the patient can be a candidate for epilepsy surgery.

REFERENCES

1. Zaporojan L, McNamara PH, Williams JA, Bergin C, Redmond J, Doherty CP. Seizures in HIV: the case for special consideration. Epilepsy Behav Case Rep. 2018;10:38-43.
2. Oshinaike O, Akinbami A, Okubadejo N, Ojo O, Ojelabi O, Dosunmu A, et al. New-Onset Seizures in HIV Patients on Antiretroviral Therapy at a Tertiary Centre in South-West, Nigeria. World J AIDS. 2013;3:67-70.
3. Siddiqi O, Birbeck GL. Safe treatment of seizures in the setting of HIV/AIDS. Curr Treat Options Neurol. 2013;15(4):529-43.
4. Sarma AK, Khandker N, Kurczewski L, Brophy GM. Medical management of epileptic seizures: challenges and solutions Neuropsychiatr Dis Treat. 2016;12:467-85.

CHAPTER 6

Management of Status Epilepticus

INTRODUCTION

Status epilepticus (SE) is a life-threatening neurologic disorder. SE can represent an exacerbation of a pre-existing seizure disorder or the initial manifestation of a seizure disorder (epilepsy) or it can represent an insult other than a seizure disorder.[1]

INVESTIGATIONS

The principal modalities, which are used in the investigation of SE, are described in **Box 1.**

Box 1 Investigations of status epilepticus.

Stat laboratory studies
- Glucose and electrolyte levels (including calcium, magnesium)
- Complete blood count
- Renal and liver function tests
- Toxicological screening and anticonvulsant drug levels
- Arterial blood gas results
- Liver function tests

Other tests that may be appropriate depending on the clinical setting
- Electroencephalography
- Blood cultures
- Urinalysis and/or cerebrospinal fluid analysis
- If a central nervous system infection is suspected, consider performing a lumbar puncture
- Imaging studies

Imaging modalities used to evaluate status epilepticus
- CT scanning and/or MRI of the brain
- Chest radiography for etiology

TREATMENT PRINCIPLES

1. Establish intravenous (IV) access, in a large vein for anticonvulsant administration because it allows therapeutic levels to be attained more rapidly.
2. Begin cardiac and other hemodynamic monitoring.
3. Ensure airway control.
4. Correct any metabolic imbalances.
5. Control hyperthermia.
6. Administer a 50 mL bolus of 50% dextrose IV and 100 mg of thiamine.
7. Give IV benzodizapines. (Followed by IV antiepilepics).
8. If seizures continue after 20 minutes, give additional fosphenytoin (10 mg PE/kg IV) or phenytoin (10 mg/kg IV). Aim for a total serum phenytoin level of about 22–25 µg/mL.
9. If seizures continue, consider administering general anesthesia with medications such as propofol, midazolam, or pentobarbital.
    - Use short-acting paralytics to ensure that ongoing seizure activity is not masked.
10. If the patient promptly becomes alert after receiving a benzodiazepine or other AED, that tends to corroborate the diagnosis of SE. The 2016 American Epilepsy Society (AES) guidelines for SE are given in **Table 1**.
    - Use electroencephalogram (EEG) monitoring if long-acting paralytics are used and if a question exists about seizure cessation.
11. In patients with epilepsy partialis continua who had been receiving antiepileptic drug (AED) treatment, knowledge of the patient's usual regimen and current levels may be pivotal. As an alternative to fosphenytoin or phenytoin, supplementation of their routine medication (guided by Stat AED levels) may help suppress their seizures.
    - Failure to respond to optimal benzodiazepine and phenytoin loading operationally defines refractory SE. If seizures continue after 20 minutes, give phenobarbital (15 mg/kg IV). Use caution when adding barbiturates to benzodiazepines because their coadministration may potentiate ventilatory failure. This may be especially true for patients (e.g., elderly patients) with impaired drug clearance.

Table 1	The 2016 American Epilepsy Society (AES) guidelines for status epilepticus (SE).[2]
Phase	**Treatment**
Stabilization phase (0–5 minutes of seizure activity)	Standard first-aid for seizures should be initiated
Initial therapy phase (5–20 minutes of seizure activity)	A benzodiazepine (specifically IM midazolam, IV lorazepam, or IV diazepam) is recommended as initial therapy
Second phase (20–40 minutes of seizure activity)	• IV fosphenytoin, valproic acid, or levetiracetam • If none of these is available, IV phenobarbital is a reasonable alternative.
Third phase (40+ minutes of seizure activity)	If a patient experiences 40+ minutes of seizure activity, treatment considerations should include repeating second-line therapy or anesthetic doses of thiopental, midazolam, pentobarbital, or propofol

(IM: intramuscular; IV: intravenous)

MANAGEMENT

The basic principles of emergency care [i.e., attention to airway, breathing, and circulation (ABCs)] apply to focal as well as to generalized SE. Aggressive treatment is required for both generalized tonic-clonic SE and subtle SE.

Management of Refractory SE and Super Refractory SE

Patients who do not recover to their baseline neurological status within 20–30 minutes of initiating therapy should undergo continuous EEG monitoring to diagnose ongoing nonconvulsive status epilepticus (NCSE). There are no evidence-based guidelines for managing refractory SE (RSE) and super refractory SE (SRSE). The treatment of RSE must be individualized to the clinical situation. Early induction of pharmacological coma has been practiced in generalized-convulsive SE using midazolam, propofol, or barbiturates. Other treatments such as inhalational anesthetic, oral antiepileptic drugs, immunomodulatory compounds, or nonpharmacological approaches (electroconvulsive treatment, hypothermia, ketogenic diet, transcranial magnetic stimulation) have been used in resistant SE. These therapies do not have randomized controlled trials and their place in therapy is yet to be established.[3]

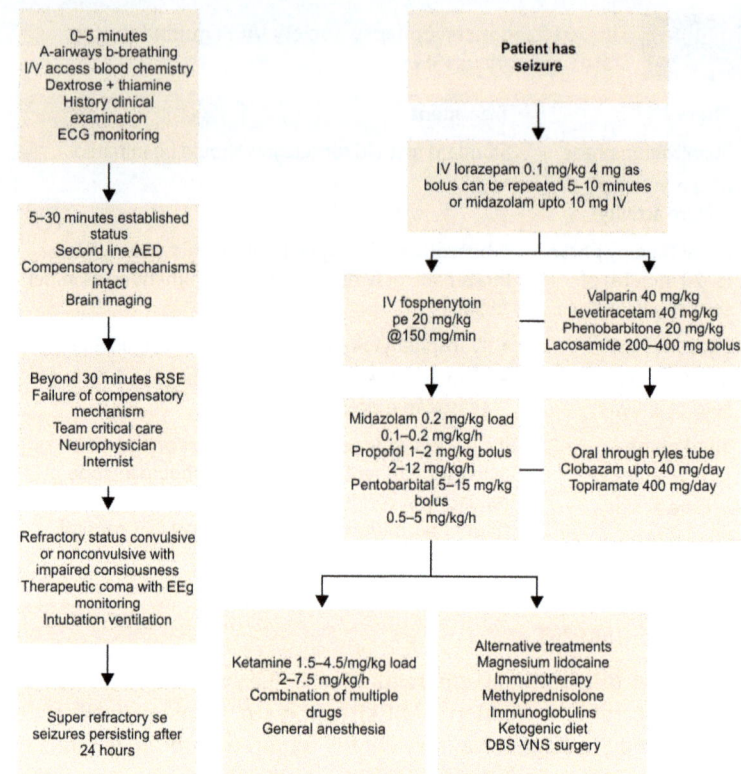

FLOWCHART 1: Management of Status Epilepticus

(AED: antiepileptic drug; DBS: deep brain stimulation; ECG: electrocardiogram; EEG: electroencephalogram; RSE: refractory status epilepticus; VNS: vagus nerve stimulation)

REFERENCES

1. Parviainen I, Uusaro A, Kalviainen R, Mervaala E, Ruokonen E. Propofol in the treatment of refractory status epilepticus. Intensive Care Med. 2006;32(7):1075-9.
2. Glauser T, Shinnar S, Gloss D, Alldredge B, Arya R, Bainbridge J, et al. Treatment of convulsive status epilepticus in children and adults: report of the Guideline Committee of the American Epilepsy Society. Epilepsy Curr. 2016;16(1):48-61.
3. Dubey D, Kalita J, Misra UK. Status epilepticus: refractory and super-refractory. Neurol India. 2017:5(7):12-7.

CHAPTER 7

Management of Post-traumatic Epilepsy

INTRODUCTION

Post-traumatic epilepsy (PTE) is a relatively underappreciated condition that can develop as a secondary consequence following traumatic brain injury (TBI).[1] TBI is commonly associated with the development of seizures and is responsible for about 20% of newly diagnosed epilepsy.[2]

Post-traumatic seizure (PTS) can be classified into early PTS (occurring within 7 days) and late PTS (occurring after 7 days of injury). The incidence of early PTS varies from 4% to 25%. Early PTS increases in patients who undergo surgical evacuation operations.

INVESTIGATIONS

The benefits of "routine" continuous electroencephalogram (cEEG) after TBI remain controversial since seizures have been identified in only 3.8% of patients of TBI who underwent routine cEEG. Computed tomography (CT) is effective for assessment of areas of brain injury in people following moderate-to-severe TBI, but not for mild TBI cases. Magnetic resonance imaging (MRI) the most sensitive investigation to detect structural brain changes and is the imaging modality of choice in people with PTE.[1,3]

MANAGEMENT OF SEIZURES POST-TRAUMATIC BRAIN INJURY

Interventions to reduce the risk of development of seizures in the immediate 7 days after the TBI have been considered to be an effective approach.[1]

The primary principles of management of the patients with moderate and severe TBI include alleviating intracranial pressure, avoiding hypotension and hypoxia.[4]

Higher remission rates and faster remission of seizures have been observed with the use of new antiepileptic drugs (AEDs) as compared to older AEDs.[5]

CLINICAL PEARLS

- The choice of AED is made based on the adverse effect profile of the drugs.
- Preventive measures:
  - Avoid sleep deprivation.
  - Avoid caffeine, alcohol, drugs of abuse.
- In adult patients with severe TBI (typically with prolonged loss of consciousness or amnesia, intracranial hematoma or brain contusion on CT scan, and/or depressed skull fracture):
  - Prophylactic treatment with phenytoin, beginning with an IV loading dose, should be initiated as soon as possible after injury to decrease the risk of PTSs occurring within the first 7 days.
  - Prophylactic treatment with phenytoin, carbamazepine, or valproate should not routinely be used beyond the first 7 days after injury to decrease the risk of PTSs occurring beyond that time.

REFERENCES

1. Piccenna L, Harris L, Hateley S, Tsang KT, Wilson M, Seemungal BM. Impact of anti-epileptic drug choice on discharge in acute traumatic brain injury patients. J Neurol. 2020.
2. Ben Shimon M, Shavit-Stein E, Altman K, Pick CG, Maggio N. Thrombin as key mediator of seizure development following traumatic brain injury. Front Pharmacol. 2020;10:1532.
3. Chen M, Edwards S, Reutens D. Complement in the development of post-traumatic epilepsy: prospects for drug repurposing. J Neurotrauma. 2020;37(5):692-705.
4. Abdelmalik PA, Draghic N, Ling GSF. Management of moderate and severe traumatic brain injury. Transfusion. 2019;59(S2):1529-38.
5. Šapina L, Ratković M. Treatment of posttraumatic epilepsy with new generation antiepileptic drugs (AEDs) - our experience. Med Glas (Zenica). 2017;14(1):126-31.

Index

Page numbers followed by *b* refer to box, and *t* refer to table.

A

American Epilepsy Society Guidelines for Status Epilepticus 23*t*
Aminophylline 15*t*
Amnesia 26
Anticonvulsant drug levels 21
Antiepileptic drugs 2, 6, 8, 11, 16*t*, 18, 19, 19*t*, 22
    specific 15
Arterial blood gas 21
Atazanavir 19*t*
Attention deficit hyperactivity disorder 2

B

Barbiturates 12
Benzodiazepine 12, 23
Beta-blockers 15*t*
Beta-lactam antibiotics isoniazid metronidazole 15*t*
Blood
    cultures 21
    urea nitrogen 14
Bone mineral density 10
Breast milk, concentrations in 11
Bupropion 15*t*

C

Calcium 13
Carbamazepine 16*t*, 19*t*, 26
Carotid doppler ultrasonography 14*t*
Catamenial epilepsy 9
Central nervous system 18
Centrotemporal spikes, benign childhood epilepsy with 2
Chlorpromazine 15*t*
Clobazam 19
Clomipramine 15*t*
Clozapine 15*t*
Cognitive impairment, migraine sleep problems 2
Complete blood count 13*t*
Continuous spike-and-wave during sleep 2
Cortical brain tumors 5, 6
Creatinine 14*t*
Cyclic antidepressants 15*t*

E

Efavirenz 19*t*
Electroencephalogram 22, 25
Electrolytes 13
Epilepsy 1, 4-6, 6*t*, 8, 13
    diagnosis of 4*t*
    juvenile
        absence 4, 6
        myoclonic 4, 6
    photosensitive 5, 6
    post-traumatic 25
    prevalence of 13
    reading 5, 6
    surgery 16
    syndromes 2*t*, 4*t*, 6*t*
        treatment for 6
    treatment for 6
    types of 9
Eslicarbazepine 10*t*

F

Felbamate 12
Fosphenytoin 23

G

Gabapentin 10*t*, 11*t*, 16*t*, 20*t*
Glucose and electrolyte levels 21
Gonadotropin-releasing hormone analogs 9

H

Hepatic function 15
Highly active antiretroviral therapy 19*t*
Holter monitoring 14*t*
Hormone replacement therapy 10
Human immunodeficiency virus
 antiepileptic drugs for 19*t*
 infection, complications of 18
Hypoxia ischemia 1

I

Intracranial hematoma 26

L

Lacosamide 10*t*, 16*t*, 20*t*
Lamotrigine 8-11, 16, 19
Landau–Kleffner syndrome 2*t*
Levetiracetam 9, 10*t*, 11*t*, 16*t*, 19*t*, 23*t*
Life-threatening neurologic disorder 21
Liver function tests 14*t*, 21*t*
Lopinavir 19*t*
Lorazepam 23*t*
Lumbar puncture 14*t*

M

Magnesium 14*t*
Maprotiline 15*t*
Medroxyprogesterone 9
Methylphenidate 15*t*

Midazolam 19*t*
Monoamine oxidase inhibitors 15

N

New antiepileptic drugs
 during pregnancy, serum concentrations of 10*t*
 use of 26
Non-nucleoside reverse transcriptase inhibitor 19

O

Olanzapine 15*t*
Oxcarbazepine 8-11, 16*t*, 19*t*
 active metabolite of 11

P

Panayiotopoulos syndrome 2
Perampanel 16
Pethidine 15*t*
Phenytoin 19*t*, 26
Phosphorus 14*t*
Plasma protein 15
Polycystic ovary syndrome 8
 incidence of 8
Pregabalin 10*t*, 16*t*, 20*t*
Progesterone 9

Q

Quetiapine 15*t*

R

Raltegravir 19*t*
Risperidone 15*t*
Ritonavir 19*t*

S

Seizures 1, 18
 benign partial 5, 6
 incidence of 18

investigation 18
management of 18
neonatal 1
post-traumatic 25
brain injury, management of 25
type, diagnosis of 20
Selective serotonin reuptake inhibitors 15
Serologic tests 14*t*
Several epilepsy syndromes 1
Sex hormones 9
Sodium valproate 9
Status epilepticus 21
investigations of 21
management of 21, 22
nonconvulsive 23
Subacute sclerosing panencephalitis 5, 6
Synthetic hormones 9

T

Theophylline 15*t*
Topiramate 10*t*, 16*t*
Toxicological screening 21*b*
Tramadol 15*t*
Traumatic brain injury 25

V

Valproate 8, 16*t*, 26
Valproic acid 19*t*, 23*t*
Vigabatrin 12

Z

Zidovudine 19*t*
Zonisamide 9, 10*t*, 11*t*, 16*t*

5217IPUKR00016B/1242
UKHW021827140426
Pitfield, Milton Keynes, MK11 3LW, UK
Ingram Content Group UK Ltd.
www.ingramcontent.com/pod-product-compliance

EU GSPR Authorised Representative
Logos Europe, 9 rue Nicolas Poussin
1700, La Rochelle, France
Phone: +33 (0) 6 67 93 73 78
E-mail: contact@logoseurope.eu